CANCER DIET COOKBOOK

28 Days Easy Breezy Nourishing Breakfast Recipes for Healing and Recovery

MAYRA N. TOVAR

In the realm of battling cancer, the significance of nutrition cannot be overstated. The food we consume plays a crucial role in supporting our bodies through the arduous journey of diagnosis, treatment, and recovery. The Cancer Diet Cookbook is a comprehensive guide that aims to empower individuals and their loved ones with knowledge and delicious recipes specifically designed to aid in healing and rejuvenation.

Throughout the pages of this book, you will find an assortment of nourishing recipes carefully curated to address the unique dietary needs and challenges faced by cancer patients. But before we delve into the wealth of culinary delights, let us share a story—a tale that embodies the transformative power of food and the hope it can instill.

Meet Emily, a vibrant and courageous soul who embarked on a life-altering battle against cancer. From the moment of her diagnosis, she confronted the disease with unwavering determination, seeking every possible means to regain control over her health and well-being. In her quest for solutions, Emily stumbled upon the Cancer Diet Cookbook, a beacon of hope amidst the storm.

As Emily delved into the pages of this invaluable resource, she discovered a treasure trove of knowledge that transcended mere recipes. The book not only offered delicious meal ideas but also provided in-depth insights into the profound connection between nutrition and cancer. It illuminated the potential of food to enhance the body's natural defense mechanisms, promote healing, and mitigate the side effects of conventional treatments.

Armed with newfound understanding, Emily embraced the principles outlined in the Cancer Diet Cookbook. She embarked on a culinary journey, exploring the vibrant world of wholesome ingredients and innovative cooking techniques. She learned to view each meal as an opportunity to nourish her body, optimize her immune system, and provide it with the strength it needed to fight back.

The recipes within the Cancer Diet Cookbook served as a lifeline for Emily. They seamlessly integrated into her daily routine, bringing joy and satisfaction to her dining experience. From vibrant salads bursting with antioxidants to comforting soups rich in healing nutrients, each recipe was meticulously crafted to strike a balance between taste and therapeutic value.

Over time, Emily noticed remarkable changes in her well-being. The fatigue that had once plagued her gradually diminished, replaced by a renewed sense of vitality. Her appetite, often suppressed by the challenges of treatment, was reignited by the flavors and textures found within these pages. And as she nourished her body with nutrient-dense meals, she witnessed a newfound resilience emerging within her.

But perhaps the most profound transformation occurred during Emily's visits to the medical facility.

Her oncologist, astounded by her progress, marveled at the positive impact of her diet on her overall health. The treatments that had once left her depleted now seemed more tolerable, with fewer side effects impeding her journey toward recovery. Emily's resilience, fortified by the nourishment she provided her body, offered a glimmer of hope in the face of adversity.

Emily's story is not an isolated incident but rather a testament to the power of food in our lives. The Cancer Diet Cookbook is here to guide you along a similar path—a path paved with knowledge, resilience, and, most importantly, nourishment. Within these pages, you will find not only recipes but also the tools to reclaim control over your health, support your body through its healing process, and embrace the joy of food as an integral part of your journey.

So, join us as we embark on a culinary expedition, celebrating the immense potential of food to aid in healing and recovery. The Cancer Diet Cookbook is more than a collection of recipes — it is a testament to the indomitable spirit that resides within each one of us, reminding us that with every bite, we have the power to nourish our bodies, revitalize our souls, and overcome the most formidable of challenges. Together, let us savor the flavors of hope and resilience.

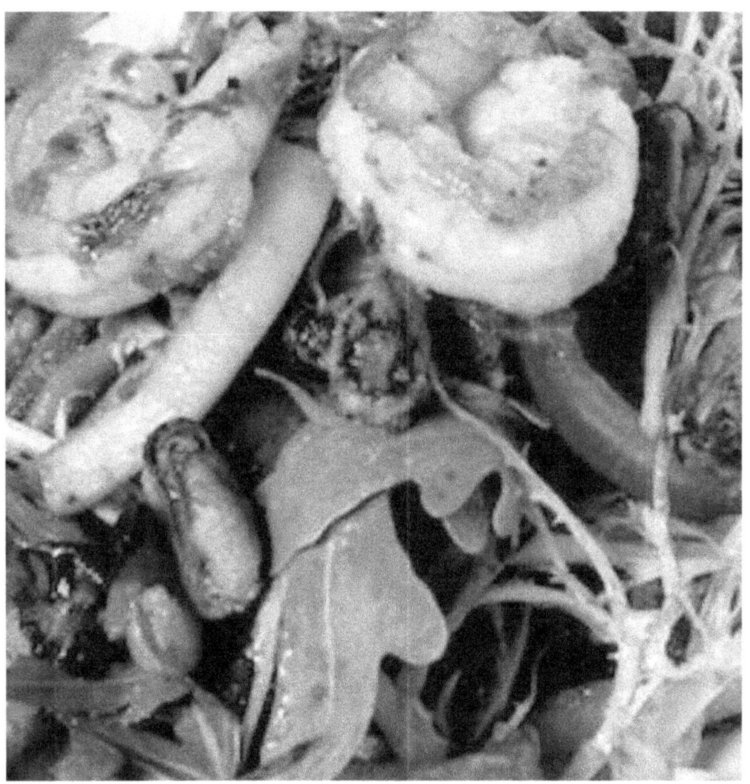

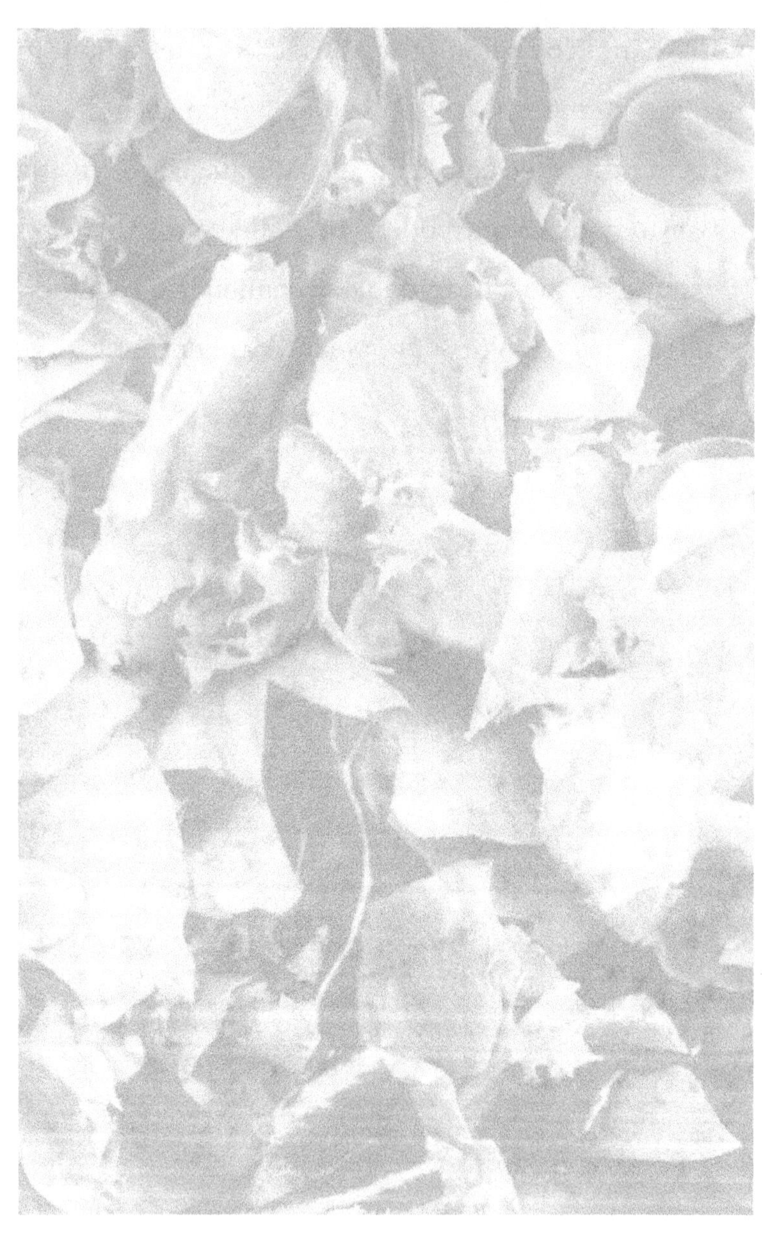

In addition to the crucial role of nutrition, easing the emotional, mental, and psychological burden of cancer requires a multifaceted approach that addresses the holistic well-being of individuals facing this challenging journey. Here are some key factors that can prove pivotal in providing support and relief during this time:

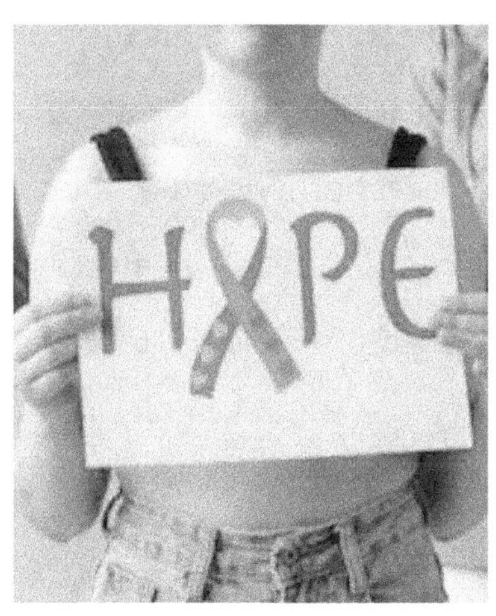

Support System: A strong support system can make a world of difference for cancer patients. Surrounding oneself with caring family members, friends, support groups, and healthcare professionals who understand and empathize with the emotional challenges of cancer can provide invaluable comfort and reassurance. Sharing experiences, seeking advice, and receiving encouragement from others who have gone through similar journeys can foster a sense of belonging and alleviate feelings of isolation.

Open Communication: Honest and open communication is essential when dealing with cancer. Encouraging individuals to express their fears, concerns, and emotions in a safe and non-judgmental environment can help alleviate the mental and emotional burden. It allows for the sharing of information, enables loved ones to provide appropriate support, and strengthens the bond between patients, caregivers, and healthcare professionals. Open communication also fosters the empowerment of patients to actively participate in their treatment decisions, giving them a sense of control and involvement.

Self-Care: Taking care of one's physical, mental, and emotional well-being is paramount during the cancer journey. Engaging in self-care activities that promote relaxation, stress reduction, and overall well-being can have a positive impact on the emotional and psychological state. This can include practices such as mindfulness, meditation, yoga, deep breathing exercises, engaging in hobbies or activities that bring joy, and prioritizing adequate rest and sleep. Nurturing oneself through self-care can help individuals better cope with the emotional challenges that cancer presents.

Mental Health Support: The emotional toll of cancer can be overwhelming, and seeking professional mental health support can be immensely beneficial. Psychologists, counselors, or therapists who specialize in oncology can provide a safe space for individuals to explore their feelings, address anxiety or depression, and develop coping strategies tailored to their specific needs. Mental health support can encompass individual counseling, support groups, or therapies such as cognitive-behavioral therapy (CBT) to help manage stress, anxiety, and depression.

Education and Empowerment: Providing individuals with access to reliable information about their diagnosis, treatment options, and potential side effects can empower them to make informed decisions and actively participate in their care. Education about cancer, its management, and available resources can help alleviate anxiety and uncertainty. Empowering individuals with knowledge equip them to ask questions, seek appropriate support, and take an active role in their physical and emotional well-being.

Emotional Expression: Encouraging individuals to express their emotions freely can be a vital aspect of coping with cancer. Whether through talking, journaling, creative expression, or engaging in support groups, giving space to emotions such as fear, anger, sadness, or frustration allows for emotional release and can foster a sense of relief and emotional well-being. Honoring and validating these emotions creates an environment where individuals can process their feelings and find strength in their vulnerability.

Lifestyle Adaptations: Making lifestyle adaptations to support mental and emotional well-being can be essential. This can involve incorporating stress management techniques, engaging in regular physical activity (as permitted by the healthcare team), maintaining a balanced diet, and avoiding unhealthy coping mechanisms such as excessive alcohol consumption or tobacco use. Small, positive changes to one's daily routine can contribute to overall well-being and resilience.

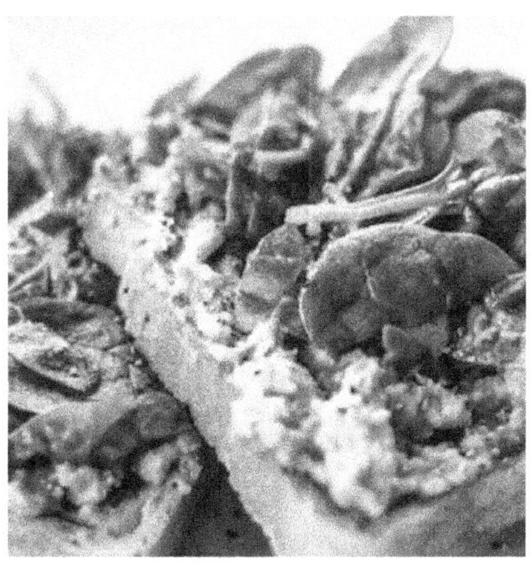

Mornings can be hectic, especially for individuals undergoing cancer treatment or in the recovery phase. Yet, starting the day with a nutritious breakfast is essential for fueling the body and setting a positive tone for the day ahead. In this section, we present a collection of easy breezy breakfast recipes specifically designed with the principles of the cancer diet in mind.

These breakfast recipes are not only delicious but also focus on incorporating nutrient-dense ingredients that can support overall health and well-being during the cancer journey. From energizing smoothies packed with antioxidants to nourishing overnight oats brimming with fiber and vital nutrients, these recipes aim to provide a satisfying and wholesome start to your day.

Whether you're seeking quick and convenient options or prefer to savor a leisurely morning meal, these easy breezy breakfast recipes are designed to fit seamlessly into your routine. Embrace the nourishing power of a well-balanced breakfast and embark on a journey of culinary delight that supports your health and enhances your vitality as you navigate through your cancer journey.

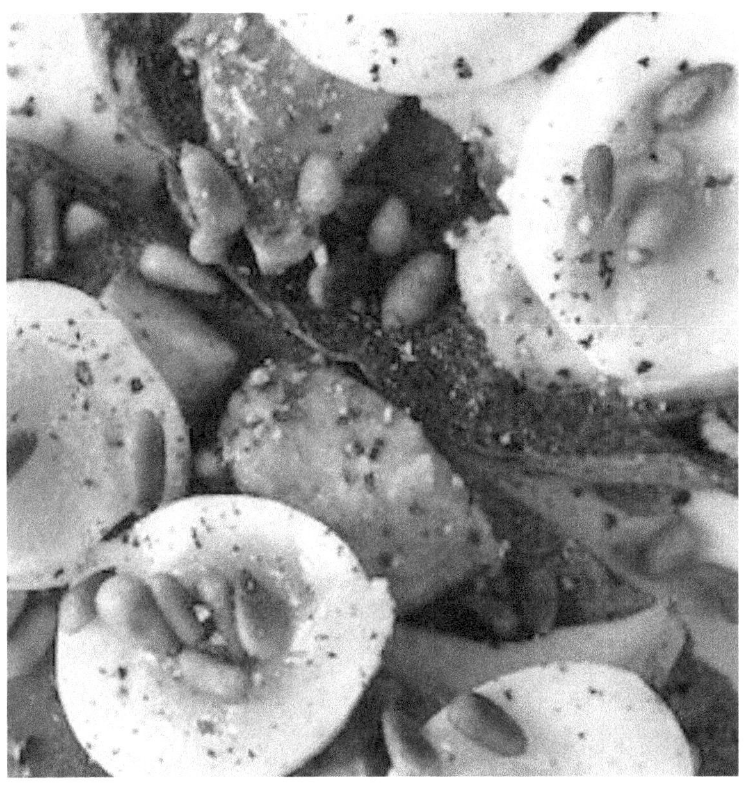

Day 1: Green Smoothie Bowl

Ingredients:

- 1 ripe banana
- 1 cup spinach
- 1/2 cup unsweetened almond milk
- 1 tablespoon chia seeds
- **Toppings**: sliced kiwi, fresh berries, shredded coconut, chopped nuts

Instructions:

1. In a blender, combine banana, spinach, almond milk, and chia seeds.
2. Blend until smooth and creamy.
3. Pour the smoothie into a bowl.
4. Top with sliced kiwi, fresh berries, shredded coconut, and chopped nuts.

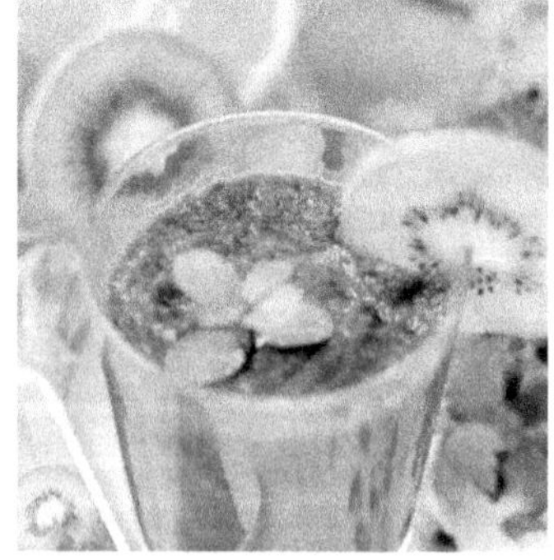

Day 2: Quinoa Breakfast Porridge

Ingredients:

- 1/2 cup cooked quinoa
- 1/2 cup unsweetened almond milk
- 1 tablespoon honey or maple syrup
- 1/4 teaspoon cinnamon

Toppings: sliced banana, chopped almonds, dried cranberries

Instructions:

1. In a saucepan, heat cooked quinoa and almond milk over medium heat.
2. Stir in honey or maple syrup and cinnamon.
3. Cook for 2-3 minutes until heated through.
4. Transfer the porridge to a bowl.
5. Top with sliced banana, chopped almonds, and dried cranberries.

Day 3: Smoked Salmon Avocado Toast

Ingredients:

- 2 slices whole grain bread, toasted
- 1/2 ripe avocado
- 1 tablespoon lemon juice
- 2 ounces of smoked salmon
- Fresh dill (optional)
- Salt and pepper to taste

Instructions:

1. In a bowl, mash the avocado with lemon juice.
2. Spread the mashed avocado evenly on the toasted bread slices.
3. Top with smoked salmon.
4. Garnish with fresh dill, if desired.
5. Season with salt and pepper to taste.

Day 4: Veggie Egg Muffins

Ingredients:

- 4 large eggs
- 1/4 cup diced bell peppers (any color)
- 1/4 cup diced zucchini
- 1/4 cup diced mushrooms
- 1/4 cup chopped spinach
- Salt and pepper to taste
- Cooking spray

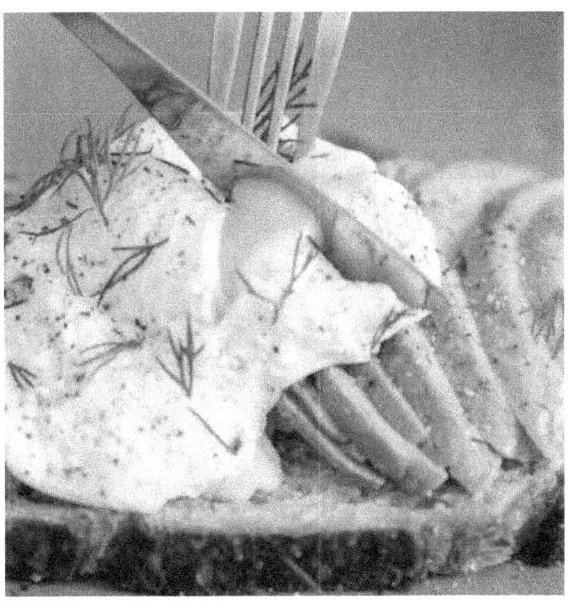

Instructions:

1. Preheat the oven to 350°F (175°C).

2. In a bowl, whisk the eggs with salt and pepper.

3. Spray a muffin tin with cooking spray.

4. Divide the diced vegetables and chopped spinach evenly among the muffin cups.

5. Pour the whisked eggs over the vegetables, filling each cup about 3/4 full.

6. Bake for 20-25 minutes until the egg muffins are set and lightly golden.

7. Allow them to cool slightly before removing from the tin.

8. Serve warm or at room temperature.

Day 5: Coconut Chia Pudding

Ingredients:

- 1/4 cup chia seeds
- 1 cup coconut milk
- 1 tablespoon honey or maple syrup
- 1/4 teaspoon vanilla extract

Toppings: fresh berries, sliced almonds, shredded coconut

Instructions:

1. In a jar or container, combine chia seeds, coconut milk, honey or maple syrup, and vanilla extract.
2. Stir well to combine.
3. Cover and refrigerate for at least 2 hours or overnight, stirring occasionally.
4. Once the chia pudding has thickened, give it a final stir.
5. Top with fresh berries, sliced almonds, and shredded coconut.

Day 6: Buckwheat Pancakes

Ingredients:

- 1 cup buckwheat flour
- 1 tablespoon baking powder
- 1 tablespoon honey or maple syrup
- 1 cup almond milk (or any milk of your choice)
- 1 large egg
- 1 tablespoon melted coconut oil

Toppings: sliced bananas, walnuts, drizzle of honey

Instructions:

1. In a bowl, whisk together buckwheat flour and baking powder.
2. In a separate bowl, whisk honey or maple syrup, almond milk, egg, and melted coconut oil.
3. Pour the wet ingredients into the dry ingredients and stir until just combined.
4. Heat a non-stick pan or griddle over medium heat.

5. Pour 1/4 cup of batter onto the pan for each pancake.

6. Cook until bubbles form on the surface, then flip and cook for another minute or until golden brown.

7. Repeat with the remaining batter.

8. Serve the buckwheat pancakes with sliced bananas, walnuts, and a drizzle of honey.

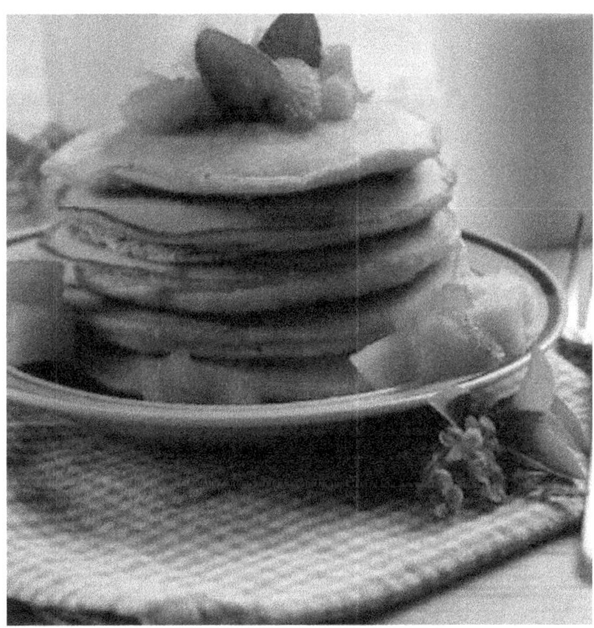

Day 7: Apple Cinnamon Overnight Oats

Ingredients:

- 1/2 cup rolled oats
- 1/2 cup unsweetened almond milk
- 1/2 cup grated apple
- 1 tablespoon honey or maple syrup
- 1/2 teaspoon cinnamon

Toppings: diced apple, raisins, chopped walnuts

Instructions:

1. In a jar or container, combine rolled oats, almond milk, grated apple, honey or maple syrup, and cinnamon.
2. Stir well to combine.
3. Cover and refrigerate overnight.
4. In the morning, give it a good stir.
5. Top with diced apples, raisins, and chopped walnuts.

Day 8: Spinach and Mushroom Frittata

Ingredients:

- 4 large eggs
- 1/4 cup diced onion
- 1/4 cup sliced mushrooms
- A handful of fresh spinach
- Salt and pepper to taste
- 1 tablespoon olive oil

Instructions:

- Preheat the oven to 350°F (175°C).
- In a bowl, whisk the eggs with salt and pepper.
- Heat olive oil in an oven-safe skillet over medium heat.
- Add the diced onion and sliced mushrooms to the skillet. Sauté until softened.
- Add the fresh spinach and cook until wilted.
- Pour the whisked eggs over the vegetables.

+ Cook for a few minutes until the edges start to set.

+ Transfer the skillet to the preheated oven and bake for about 10 minutes or until the frittata is set in the center.

+ Remove from the oven and let it cool slightly before slicing.

+ Serve warm or at room temperature.

+ Enjoy this protein-packed spinach and mushroom frittata.

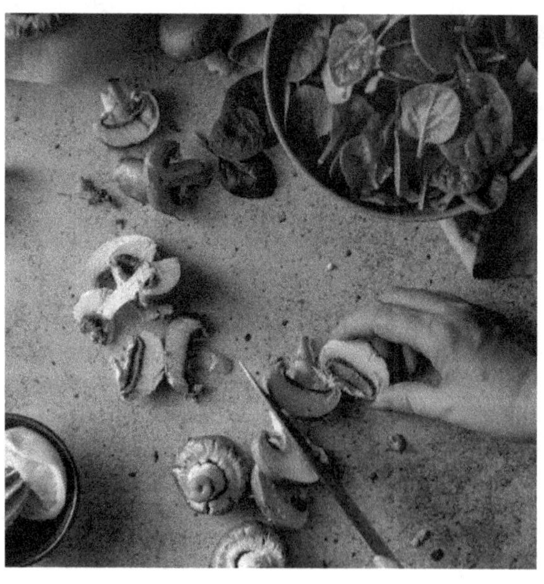

Day 9: Peanut Butter Banana Toast

Ingredients:

- 2 slices whole grain bread, toasted
- 2 tablespoons natural peanut butter
- 1 ripe banana, sliced
- 1 tablespoon chia seeds (optional)
- Drizzle of honey (optional)

Instructions:

1. Spread peanut butter evenly on the toasted bread slices.
2. Top with sliced banana.
3. Sprinkle with chia seeds, if desired.
4. Drizzle with honey for added sweetness, if desired.

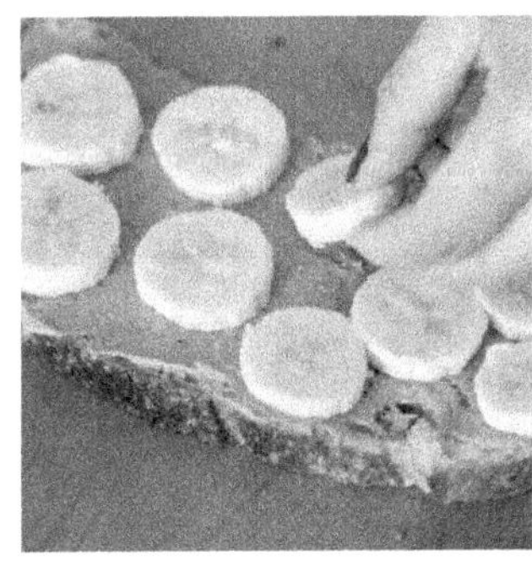

Day 10: Vegetable Breakfast Burrito

Ingredients:

- 1 large tortilla wrap
- 2 eggs, beaten
- 1/4 cup diced bell peppers (any color)
- 1/4 cup diced zucchini
- 1/4 cup diced tomatoes
- Handful of fresh spinach
- Salt and pepper to taste
- 1 tablespoon olive oil
- Salsa or hot sauce (optional)

Instructions:

1. Heat olive oil in a skillet over medium heat.
2. Add diced bell peppers, zucchini, and tomatoes to the skillet. Sauté until softened.
3. Add fresh spinach and cook until wilted.
4. Pour the beaten eggs into the skillet with the vegetables.

5. Cook, stirring occasionally, until the eggs are scrambled and cooked to your liking.

6. Season with salt and pepper.

7. Warm the tortilla wrap in a separate pan or microwave for a few seconds.

8. Place the scrambled eggs and vegetable mixture onto the tortilla.

Optional: Serve with salsa or hot sauce on the side.

Roll up the tortilla, tucking in the sides as you go.

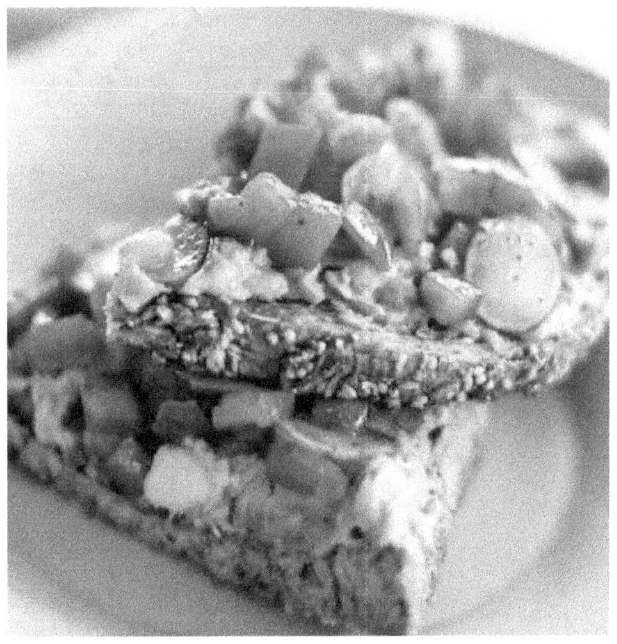

Day 11: Acai Bowl

Ingredients:

- 1 pack frozen acai puree (unsweetened)
- 1/2 ripe banana
- 1/4 cup unsweetened almond milk

Toppings: sliced banana, granola, coconut flakes, chia seeds

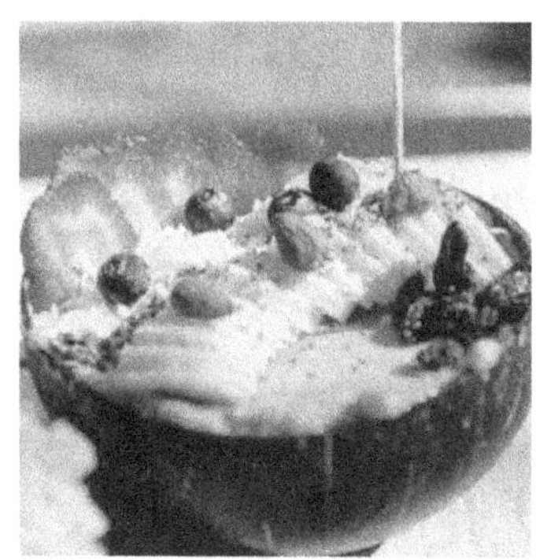

Instructions:

1. In a blender, combine frozen acai puree, ripe banana, and almond milk.
2. Blend until smooth and creamy.
3. Pour the acai mixture into a bowl.
4. Top with sliced banana, granola, coconut flakes, and chia seeds.

Day 12: Sweet Potato Toast with Almond Butter

Ingredients:

- 1 large sweet potato
- Natural almond butter

Toppings: sliced strawberries, crushed almonds, drizzle of honey

Instructions:

1. Slice the sweet potato lengthwise into 1/4-inch-thick slices.
2. Toast the sweet potato slices in a toaster or toaster oven until tender.
3. Spread almond butter generously on each sweet potato slice.
4. Top with sliced strawberries, crushed almonds, and a drizzle of honey.

Day 13: Berry Chia Jam on Whole Grain Toast

Ingredients:

- 1 cup mixed berries (strawberries, blueberries, raspberries)
- 1 tablespoon chia seeds
- 1 tablespoon honey or maple syrup
- 2 slices whole grain bread, toasted

Instructions:

1. In a small saucepan, combine mixed berries, chia seeds, and honey or maple syrup.
2. Cook over medium heat, stirring occasionally, until the berries soften and release their juices.
3. Mash the berries with a fork or potato masher to desired consistency.
4. Remove from heat and let the chia jam cool and thicken.
5. Spread the chia jam on the toasted whole grain bread slices.

Day 14: Turmeric Oatmeal with Almonds

Ingredients:

- 1/2 cup rolled oats
- 1 cup unsweetened almond milk
- 1/2 teaspoon ground turmeric
- 1/4 teaspoon ground cinnamon
- 1 tablespoon honey or maple syrup
- Handful of almonds, chopped

Instructions:

1. In a saucepan, combine rolled oats, almond milk, turmeric, cinnamon, and honey or maple syrup.
2. Stir well to combine.
3. Cook over medium heat, stirring occasionally, until the oats are cooked and the mixture thickens.
4. Remove from heat and let it cool slightly.
5. Top with chopped almonds.

Day 15: Avocado and Tomato Toast

Ingredients:

- 2 slices whole grain bread, toasted
- 1 ripe avocado, sliced or mashed
- 1 ripe tomato, sliced
- Fresh basil leaves
- Salt and pepper to taste

Instructions:

1. Spread avocado evenly on the toasted bread slices.
2. Top with sliced tomato.
3. Season with salt and pepper.
4. Garnish with fresh basil leaves.

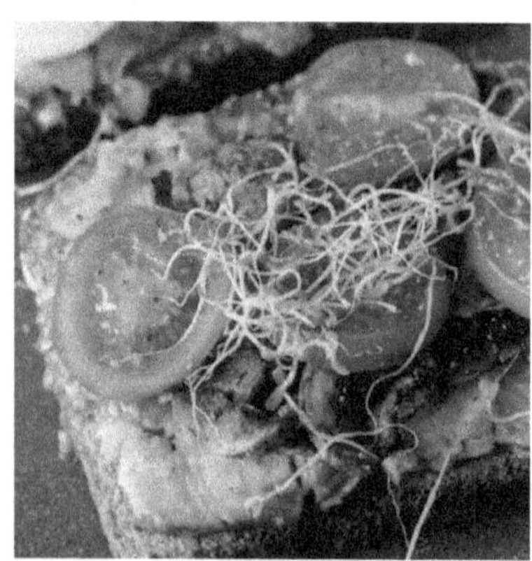

Day 16: Blueberry Protein Smoothie

Ingredients:

- 1 cup unsweetened almond milk
- 1/2 cup frozen blueberries
- 1/2 ripe banana
- 1 scoop vanilla protein powder
- 1 tablespoon almond butter
- 1 tablespoon chia seeds (optional)

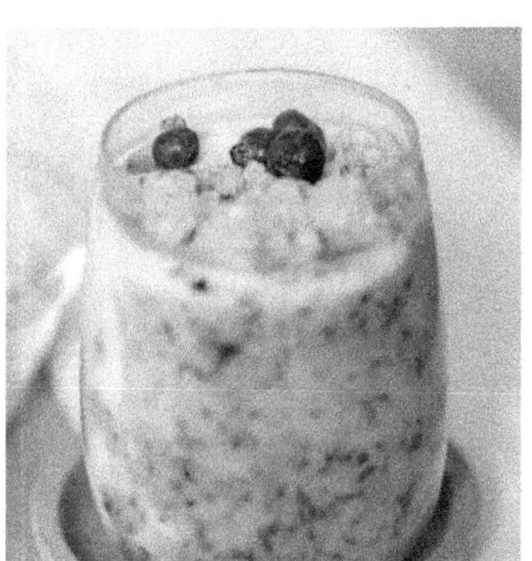

Instructions:

1. In a blender, combine almond milk, frozen blueberries, ripe banana, vanilla protein powder, almond butter, and chia seeds.
2. Blend until smooth and creamy.
3. Pour the smoothie into a glass.

Day 17: Vegetable Omelette

Ingredients:

- 2 large eggs
- 1/4 cup diced bell peppers (any color)
- 1/4 cup diced zucchini
- 1/4 cup diced tomatoes
- A handful of fresh spinach
- Salt and pepper to taste
- 1 tablespoon olive oil

Instructions:

1. In a bowl, whisk the eggs with salt and pepper.
2. Heat olive oil in a skillet over medium heat.
3. Add diced bell peppers, zucchini, and tomatoes to the skillet. Sauté until softened.
4. Add fresh spinach and cook until wilted.
5. Pour the whisked eggs into the skillet with the vegetables.

6. Cook, gently lifting the edges and tilting the skillet to let the uncooked eggs flow underneath.

7. Once the eggs are mostly set, fold the omelette in half.

8. Continue cooking for another minute until the eggs are fully cooked.

9. Transfer the omelette to a plate and let it cool slightly before serving.

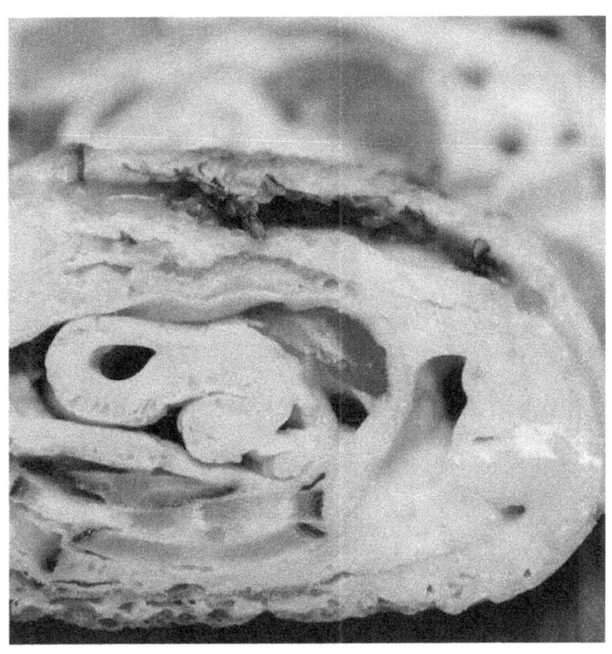

Day 18: Buckwheat Granola with Yogurt

Ingredients:

- 1 cup buckwheat groats
- 1/4 cup unsweetened shredded coconut
- 1/4 cup chopped almonds
- 1/4 cup dried cranberries
- 2 tablespoons maple syrup
- 1 tablespoon melted coconut oil
- 1/2 teaspoon vanilla extract
- Greek yogurt (or any yogurt of your choice)
- Fresh berries for topping

Instructions:

1. Preheat the oven to 325°F (160°C) and line a baking sheet with parchment paper.
2. In a bowl, combine buckwheat groats, shredded coconut, chopped almonds, and dried cranberries.

3. In a separate bowl, whisk together maple syrup, melted coconut oil, and vanilla extract.

4. Pour the wet mixture over the dry ingredients and mix well to coat.

5. Spread the mixture evenly on the prepared baking sheet.

6. Bake for 20-25 minutes, stirring occasionally, until the granola is golden brown and crispy.

7. Remove from the oven and let it cool completely.

8. Serve the buckwheat granola with yogurt and top with fresh berries.

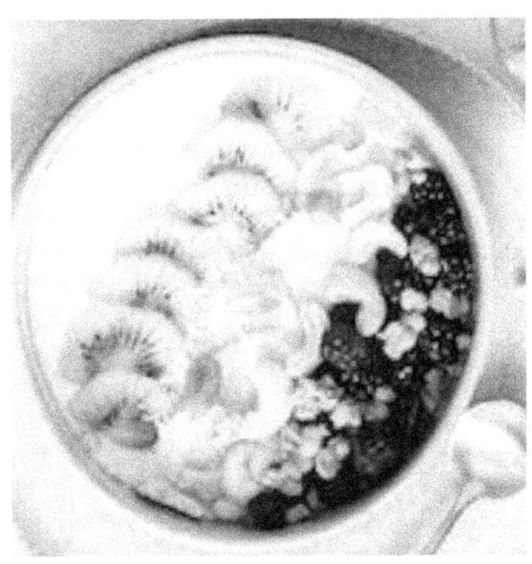

Day 19: Strawberry Banana Protein Smoothie Bowl

Ingredients:

- 1 ripe banana
- 1 cup frozen strawberries
- 1/2 cup unsweetened almond milk
- 1 scoop vanilla protein powder
- Toppings: sliced banana, fresh strawberries, granola, shredded coconut

Instructions:

1. In a blender, combine ripe bananas, frozen strawberries, almond milk, and vanilla protein powder.
2. Blend until smooth and creamy.
3. Pour the smoothie into a bowl.
4. Top with sliced banana, fresh strawberries, granola, and shredded coconut.

Day 20: Veggie Breakfast Wrap

Ingredients:

- 1 large whole wheat or spinach tortilla wrap
- 2 eggs, beaten
- 1/4 cup diced bell peppers (any color)
- 1/4 cup diced zucchini
- 1/4 cup diced tomatoes
- A handful of fresh spinach
- Salt and pepper to taste
- 1 tablespoon olive oil
- Salsa or hot sauce (optional)

Instructions:

1. Heat olive oil in a skillet over medium heat.
2. Add diced bell peppers, zucchini, and tomatoes to the skillet. Sauté until softened.
3. Add fresh spinach and cook until wilted.
4. Pour the beaten eggs into the skillet with the vegetables.

5. Cook, stirring occasionally, until the eggs are scrambled and cooked to your liking.

6. Season with salt and pepper.

7. Warm the tortilla wrap in a separate pan or microwave for a few seconds.

8. Place the scrambled eggs and vegetable mixture onto the tortilla.

9. Optional: Serve with salsa or hot sauce on the side.

10. Roll up the tortilla, tucking in the sides as you go.

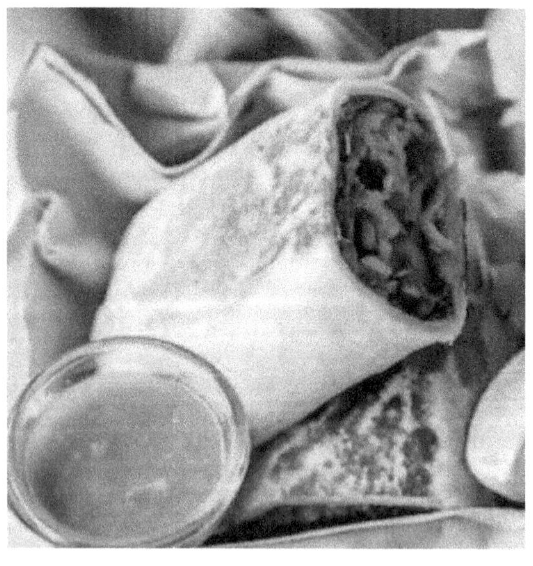

Day 21: Matcha Chia Pudding

Ingredients:

- 1/4 cup chia seeds
- 1 cup almond milk (or any milk of your choice)
- 1 tablespoon honey or maple syrup
- 1 teaspoon matcha powder

Toppings: sliced strawberries, sliced almonds, coconut flakes

Instructions:

1. In a jar or container, combine chia seeds, almond milk, honey or maple syrup, and matcha powder.
2. Stir well to combine.
3. Cover and refrigerate for at least 2 hours or overnight, stirring occasionally.
4. Once the chia pudding has thickened, give it a final stir.
5. Top with sliced strawberries, sliced almonds, and coconut flakes.

Day 22: Greek Yogurt Parfait

Ingredients:

- 1 cup Greek yogurt
- 1/4 cup granola
- 1/4 cup mixed berries (strawberries, blueberries, raspberries)
- 1 tablespoon honey or maple syrup

Instructions:

1. In a glass or jar, layer Greek yogurt, granola, and mixed berries.
2. Drizzle honey or maple syrup over the top.
3. Repeat the layers if desired.

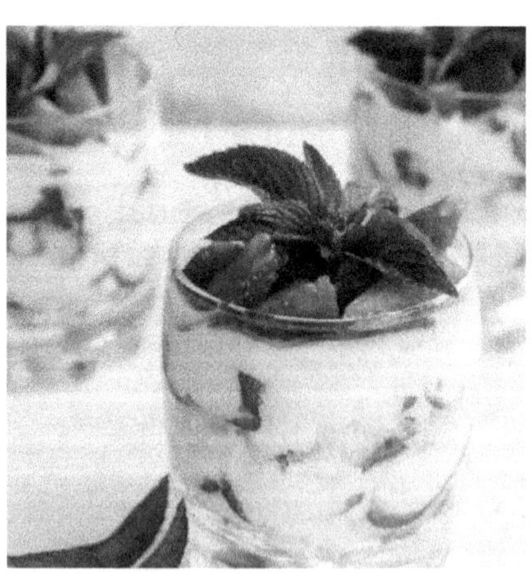

Day 23: Buckwheat Banana Bread

Ingredients:

- 1 cup buckwheat flour
- 1/2 cup almond flour
- 1 teaspoon baking powder
- 1/2 teaspoon baking soda
- 1/4 teaspoon salt
- 2 ripe bananas, mashed
- 1/4 cup honey or maple syrup
- 1/4 cup unsweetened applesauce
- 1/4 cup almond milk (or any milk of your choice)
- 1 teaspoon vanilla extract

Optional add-ins: chopped nuts, dried fruits, chocolate chips

Instructions:

1. Preheat the oven to 350°F (175°C) and grease a loaf pan.

2. In a bowl, whisk together buckwheat flour, almond flour, baking powder, baking soda, and salt.

3. In a separate bowl, mix mashed bananas, honey or maple syrup, applesauce, almond milk, and vanilla extract.

4. Pour the wet ingredients into the dry ingredients and stir until just combined.

5. If using, fold in the optional add-ins.

6. Pour the batter into the greased loaf pan.

7. Bake for 45-50 minutes or until a toothpick inserted into the center comes out clean.

8. Remove from the oven and let it cool in the pan for 10 minutes.

9. Transfer the banana bread to a wire rack and let it cool completely before slicing.

Day 24: Quinoa Breakfast Bowl

Ingredients:

- 1/2 cup cooked quinoa
- 1/4 cup unsweetened almond milk
- 1 tablespoon honey or maple syrup
- 1/2 teaspoon ground cinnamon

Toppings: sliced banana, chopped nuts, dried fruits, drizzle of honey

Instructions:

1. In a saucepan, heat cooked quinoa with almond milk, honey or maple syrup, and ground cinnamon.
2. Stir well to combine and cook until heated through.
3. Transfer the quinoa mixture to a bowl.
4. Top with sliced banana, chopped nuts, dried fruits, and a drizzle of honey.

Day 25: Green Smoothie Bowl

Ingredients:

- 1 ripe banana
- 1 cup fresh spinach
- 1/2 cup unsweetened almond milk
- 1 tablespoon almond butter

Toppings: sliced kiwi, fresh berries, granola, chia seeds

Instructions:

1. In a blender, combine ripe banana, fresh spinach, almond milk, and almond butter.
2. Blend until smooth and creamy.
3. Pour the smoothie into a bowl.
4. Top with sliced kiwi, fresh berries, granola, and chia seeds.

Day 26: Scrambled Tofu Breakfast Wrap

Ingredients:

- 1/2 block firm tofu, crumbled
- 1/4 cup diced bell peppers (any color)
- 1/4 cup diced zucchini
- 1/4 cup diced tomatoes
- Handful of fresh spinach
- 1/2 teaspoon turmeric powder
- 1/2 teaspoon garlic powder
- Salt and pepper to taste
- 1 tablespoon olive oil
- 1 large whole wheat or spinach tortilla wrap

Instructions:

1. Heat olive oil in a skillet over medium heat.
2. Add crumbled tofu, diced bell peppers, zucchini, and tomatoes to the skillet. Sauté until the vegetables are softened.
3. Add fresh spinach and cook until wilted.

4. Sprinkle turmeric powder, garlic powder, salt, and pepper over the tofu mixture. Stir well to combine and cook for another minute.

5. Warm the tortilla wrap in a separate pan or microwave for a few seconds.

6. Place the scrambled tofu mixture onto the tortilla.

7. Roll up the tortilla, tucking in the sides as you go.

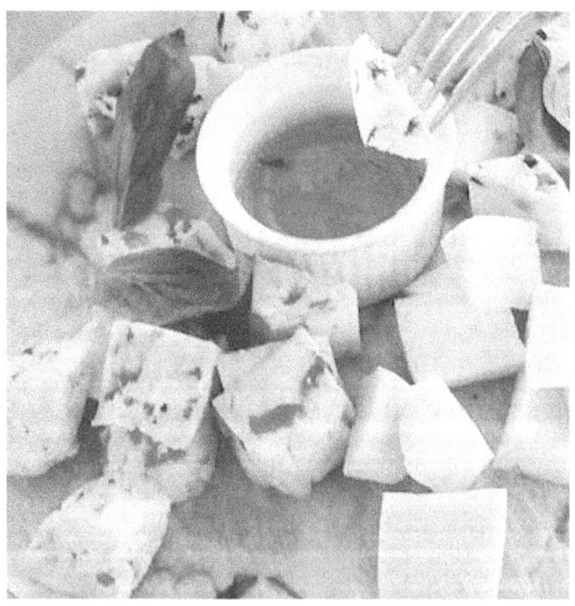

Day 27: Berry Quinoa Smoothie

Ingredients:

- 1/2 cup cooked quinoa
- 1 cup mixed berries (strawberries, blueberries, raspberries)
- 1/2 ripe banana
- 1 cup unsweetened almond milk
- 1 tablespoon honey or maple syrup

Instructions:

1. In a blender, combine cooked quinoa, mixed berries, ripe banana, almond milk, and honey or maple syrup.
2. Blend until smooth and creamy.
3. Pour the smoothie into a glass.

Day 28: Chia Seed Pudding with Fresh Fruit

Ingredients:

- 1/4 cup chia seeds
- 1 cup unsweetened almond milk
- 1 tablespoon honey or maple syrup
- 1/2 teaspoon vanilla extract

Toppings: fresh fruit (such as sliced mango, berries, or kiwi)

Instructions:

1. In a jar or container, combine chia seeds, almond milk, honey or maple syrup, and vanilla extract.
2. Stir well to combine.
3. Cover and refrigerate for at least 2 hours or overnight, stirring occasionally.
4. Once the chia pudding has thickened, give it a final stir.
5. Top with fresh fruit of your choice.

CONCLUSION

In conclusion, the Cancer Diet Cookbook offers a comprehensive collection of 28 nutritious and delicious breakfast recipes that are specifically designed to support individuals dealing with cancer. By incorporating these recipes into their daily routine, readers can take a proactive approach to their health and well-being.

The power of food in cancer management cannot be underestimated. Each recipe in this cookbook is carefully crafted to provide essential nutrients, antioxidants, and anti-inflammatory properties that can help support the body's immune system, promote healing, and boost overall health. From comforting oatmeal infused with turmeric to protein-packed smoothie bowls bursting with fresh fruits, every recipe is thoughtfully designed to provide nourishment and pleasure.

Moreover, this cookbook emphasizes the importance of a holistic approach to cancer care. It recognizes that addressing the emotional, mental, and psychological burden of cancer is just as crucial as addressing the physical aspects. The inclusion of factors such as a strong support system, open communication, and self-care highlights the significance of emotional well-being in the journey toward healing.

By following the recipes and implementing the suggested strategies, individuals can not only nourish their bodies but also find solace in taking charge of their health. The Cancer Diet Cookbook empowers readers to make informed dietary choices and provides a source of inspiration and hope as they navigate their own unique cancer journey.

It is important to note that this cookbook is not a substitute for medical advice or treatment. Individuals should always consult with their healthcare professionals or registered dietitians for personalized dietary recommendations based on their specific health conditions and dietary needs.

In closing, the Cancer Diet Cookbook serves as a valuable resource for individuals seeking guidance on nourishing their bodies during cancer treatment and beyond. Through the power of wholesome and delicious recipes, it inspires readers to embrace a cancer-fighting lifestyle and take control of their well-being. Let this cookbook be a companion on your path to better health, empowering you to make positive changes and savor each nourishing bite along the way.